does YOUR pain get in the way?

How long
have you suffered already?

How much longer
will you continue to suffer?

What do you fear
from more and more drugs?

What do you fear
from surgery … *again*?

You want more than answers –
you want relief!

We're ready to help you *right now:*
DIAL 1-800-FIX-PAIN

More life-saving treatments from best-selling author
John Parks Trowbridge M. D., FACAM

When life is your choice, failure is not an option.[SM]

I need to share this booklet right now with ...

_____

_____

_____

_____

_____

Questions I want to ask so I can get relief:

_____

_____

_____

_____

_____

_____

_____

_____

When life is your choice, failure is not an option.℠

Find it *now* – Fix it *right!*

Failure is *not* an Option

Because *health* is your greatest *wealth!*   3

When life is your choice, failure is not an option.^{SM}

Find it *now* – Fix it *right!*

Ask Rick

Rick was happy with the prolotherapy injections helping his knee. A natural solution placed into his injured tissues stimulated regrowth, repairing the damage and resulting arthritis. He asked about treating his hip. When a quarterback in high school, an onrushing opponent "nailed" his right hip with his helmet. White-lightning pain! Then lingering pains and limitations for *40 years*. I explained, "I would like to try a new and unique 'cellular allograft' ("stem cells") preparation that I think might help." Injection of this newly-developed product into his hip was easy and his hip pains disappeared quickly. Where the helmet hit was far different and much more serious, a tissue compression injury (RSD) … and *that* special pain took a whole week to disappear.

Six months later, he stepped backwards off his hay-baler (*oops* – no step there!) and fell onto – you guessed it! – his right hip. Days later he came in: "This hurts like before; should we try more cells?" "*Wait!* – this is a separate new injury. Let's see how you recover. Assuming all goes well, that's confirmation that your earlier treatment was a success." His *new* injury pains *disappeared in a week*, and he continues to comfortably enjoy usual activities like he had *never* seen in his adult years.

"Growing up" involves uncountable bumps and bruises, sometimes even breaks. We rarely understand how these often innocent events can lead to pain that arises anytime later and can last for years, even the rest of our life.

Natural healing produced by an advanced, unique "stem cell" preparation has the potential to restore greater comfort and better function for all joints, tendons, rotator cuff and other strains, back and neck pains, and other support tissues all over. This booklet shares the basic ideas you want to learn.

This illustration shows what you will learn and understand in the following pages.

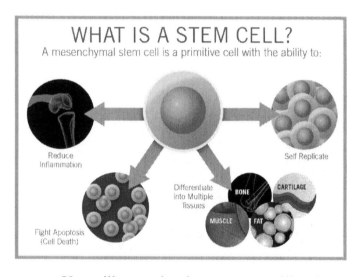

WHAT IS A STEM CELL?
A mesenchymal stem cell is a primitive cell with the ability to:

Reduce Inflammation

Self Replicate

Differentiate into Multiple Tissues

BONE

CARTILAGE

MUSCLE

FAT

Fight Apoptosis (Cell Death)

You will appreciate how easy we will make these ideas for you to understand – and then you will confidently expect our unique "stem cell" treatments to help you feel better. Honestly, you've suffered enough already.

When life is your choice, failure is not an option.℠

Find it *now* – Fix it ***right!***

Don't Confuse Me With Words!

Here I use <stem cell> to review the general topic of these cells and "stem cell" (in quotes) to refer to the highly specialized, unique, patented product that we use.

As variations on so-called <stem cell> treatments eventually become more mainstream, just *what* they are and *how* they heal is important to understand, to best treat your degenerative diseases. When special "*allo*graft" stem cell tissues (*not your own*) are used, the source *must* be a trusted one: a federally-registered tissue bank is the only one I depend on, exceeding my expectations in how these youthful cells are isolated, processed, and safely preserved.

I routinely witness impressive results "all over" … not just for my patients but also for *me*, personally. This rich source of young cells and essential growth factors ["cytokines" and "exosomes" for you Dr. Google fans to look up] promotes regeneration of joint support tissues and reduces inflammation. I nickname this patented unique preparation as "the package that performs." *Because it does!*

The term <stem cells> is recognized all over the world but it can mean *many* different things. The National Institutes of Health (NIH) describes their remarkable potential to develop into many different cell types in your body. They can serve as an internal repair system in many tissues, dividing to replenish other cells as long as you are alive.

Each <stem cell> has the ability to make *more* <stem cells> *or* to become another developed tissue cell with more specialized functions in your organs. A "bad rap" on <stem cells> arose 2 dozen years ago when people realized that embryo (developing baby) cells were being used for research; *that* practice was abruptly outlawed.

Today, most treatments elsewhere involve harvesting some of your cells by sucking fat from your belly, your butt, or your bone marrow. Then some obscure and often non-standard processing is performed on this "soup" solution, to separate your stem cells from the others *also* removed. You can see the limitations easily: a meager number of <stem cells> can be retrieved; others (such as unwanted red and white blood cells) commonly are blended in the final "soup" solution; in-office procedures might use chemicals that needlessly injure or kill some of your cells; **and** … *perhaps this is most important*: your harvested cells are "adult" stem cells, they are *already old* (your age!) and they have been *exposed* to all the toxic chemicals and heavy metals seen by your body as well as stresses and nutritional deficiencies that have been reducing optimal performance throughout *all* of your tissues.

A couple of other questions deserve to be asked regarding your *harvested* stem cells: since these cells have been inside you "forever," why haven't they *already kicked into gear* and performed needed repairs? And … could some of your stem cells be affected by illnesses brewing inside you, so they might never work as well as before?

Find it *now* – Fix it *right!*

Here's why *our* "stem cell" product is the "crown jewel" of all available stem cell options: these are obtained from pregnant American women who volunteer to donate the umbilical cord blood that would otherwise be discarded at the time of their scheduled C-section delivery (surgically removing the baby through her belly). All donors undergo extensive questioning and testing merely to qualify for donation. While every medical treatment can involve risks, *tissue banks* that comply with (or even exceed) stringent federal regulations diligently focus on excluding all foreseeable complications.

Comprehensive studies are performed on the cord blood while cells are being processed, isolated, and gently preserved by a patented process to preserve maximum survival and activity (specific cell populations with cell growth factors).

This resulting priceless "stem cell" solution is quarantined until all tests score an "A-plus" for safety and durability. Carefully measured concentrated cells are deep frozen until ordered and sent overnight to our office on dry ice, to be gently thawed only when you are ready for your treatment.

We call our treatment "stem cells" (*in quotes*, meaning the solution is composed of selected cells and critical growth factors) to identify them from the *unknown* stem cell solutions that might be severely compromised when harvested, filtered, and processed in private offices.

Umbilical cord cells are considered pluripotent, meaning they reproduce to make more robust cells *just like themselves* or they can differentiate (change into) *many specific tissue cells* in the right circumstances. Your own "adult" stem cells might already have become *limited* in the changes they can undergo to help your healing.

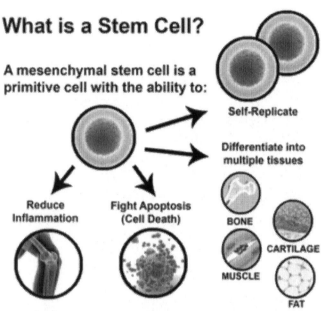

What is a Stem Cell?

A mesenchymal stem cell is a primitive cell with the ability to:

Self-Replicate

Differentiate into multiple tissues

BONE

CARTILAGE

MUSCLE

FAT

Reduce Inflammation

Fight Apoptosis (Cell Death)

Adult stem cells are the means by which our bodies naturally heal throughout our lifetime

Here's a confusing term: *mesenchymal* stem cells. Carefully isolated from umbilical cord blood, these mesenchymal cells expect to differentiate into structural support cells – helping to repair painful injured joints, arthritis, even fractured bones and other structural tissues.

Find it *now* – Fix it *right!*

Research into their possible changes into *other* specific cell types is promising but still requires more study. Remember: we simply say that our "stem cell" treatment holds the hope that you will become more comfortable and capable *but* the results seen by any one patient cannot be predicted with certainty.

Should you trust the safety and purity of these uniquely prepared "stem cells"? You can feel confident when realizing that I personally have had several of these treatments to reduce pains and limitations due to lifelong disabilities from a genetic condition related to scoliosis and double-jointedness. [Ehlers-Danlos Syndrome, for you Dr. Google fans]

One more point to consider: I took a 2-day trip to tour the laboratory facility, to meet with their Ph.D. research scientists, and to sit one-on-one with their quality control and regulatory compliance officers and their chief executive. They do it right, even more than right.

Sufficiently convinced of their long-term safety for *me*, I can say without any reservation that I am thrilled to enjoy better comfort and capability, miracles for which I have long prayed as I have grown older.

The results our patients enjoy – and *I* enjoy as well – have been truly amazing, beyond what I ever expected to see. *Our* "stem cell" solution deserves the nickname of "*the package that performs!*"

When life is your choice, failure is not an option.℠

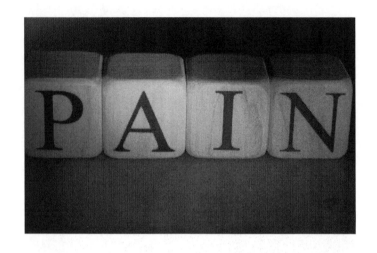

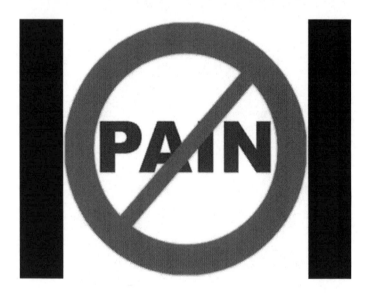

Find it *now* – Fix it *right!*

Ask Lois

Lois has spent years standing on her feet, teaching students. When not at work, she has devoted many joyful hours assisting her mother and other family members less able to fend for themselves. Over time, daily life wear and tear takes its toll in daily comfort, a situation that so many people understand. Such suffering, though, is done "in private" for the long hours as we go about our chores and duties and in the quiet of night.

Falls and crashes create lingering suffering, and Lois was amazed when she realized that discomfort from 18 earlier broken bones is now much less painful after her special "stem cells" injection. When she stood up immediately after her treatment, she noticed she was walking more easily and with a better gait. She now walks longer distances without having to rest her back *and* her arthritis overall doesn't bother her like before. Better walking means stable, safer balance.

Can our "stem cells" help all over? Well, Lois says she can get more exercise without pain like before. Is her metabolism better? She notes that she has been able to lose weight more easily – and with her recent changes, her double chin has tightened up. Oddly enough, she claims her hearing seems improved (turning down the radio volume) … maybe she's just paying more attention to life?

Remember when most of your days consisted of play?

"Let's go swimming" –

"No, I'd rather play baseball" –

"But I want to ride bikes" –

"Hey – let's do all three!"

Back then, your body wasn't the limiting factor, bumps and bruises and painful problems resolved quickly – then you were outside for more fun.

So ... how much fun is it to finally get going again with enjoyable activities? Get to feeling better, go join your friends, and find out!

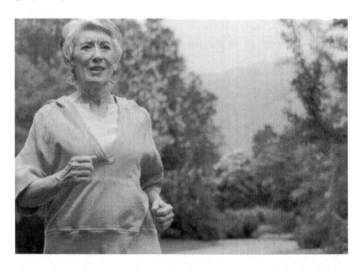

(Not into walking or running or whatever? You're old enough to break all the rules! Do something else!)

When life is your choice, failure is not an option.[SM]

Simple Simon Says … Mother, May I?

So … what if your doctor disapproves or discourages your seeking pain relief and better function from our "stem cells"?

Well, he or she might know next to nothing about this whole field of regenerative medicine, truly a practice with its own tools and expertise, where treatments are aimed at replacing or repairing damaged tissue to restore more normal function. Few doctors have invested the time and study to become recognized as experts in restoring better health. So … are you willing to bet your future on flimsy advice? If your doctoring has been so great already, then why are you *still* suffering?

What if your insurance company refuses to cover your treatment? You can absolutely count on that! **Medical** care coverage is like fire insurance for your home: you want to have it but never use it. But you want to benefit from drugs and surgery if that is what you *need* to "manage" your condition.

Something you can choose instead is totally different: **health** care. First, your doctors are trained in *illness* care and a shocking few have any training and experience in helping you go beyond fancy Band-aids to "control" your symptoms. Natural treatments can help you recover more robust, youthful, and vital capabilities you might have feared were lost forever. You guessed it: *medical* insurance does **not** cover *health* recovery programs.

What most patients – and their doctors! – fail to understand is that *real* care is more than just caring and prescribing drugs to suppress symptoms. What is easy to see is that illnesses "come on" and injuries happen "suddenly" – so these situations attract attention.

What is harder to appreciate is that "stuck" inflammation is creating virtually all discomforts and diseases: *all* aging is a **disease** happening one day at a time. What is needed (for **all** "mental" *and* physical problems) is targeting the **cause** of the problem.

Failing organ functions with sports injuries and arthritis, diabetes, cancer, headaches, chronic sinus and lung infections, high blood pressure, congestive heart failure, blocking arteries, macular degeneration vision changes, sleep apnea, gum inflammation and degenerated teeth, dysfunctional mouth ("jaws too small for your tongue"), even "trivial" constipation, "heartburn" / reflux, and a *zillion* other afflictions often go poorly treated (usually *missed*) due to overlooking the root causes.

Even more difficult for doctors and patients to understand are the subtle changes from influences in our environment that degrade our functions. When your body is impaired, inflammation persists – that is, pain continues because injured joints and other tissues cannot complete their healing and repair process.

Personal pollution by toxic metals over a lifetime is stealthy and goes undiscovered, undiagnosed, and untreated because conventional

Find it *now* – Fix it ***right!***

doctors stop asking *"Why?"* about 5 questions too soon. Drugs are "stoppers" or "blockers" (*anti*-histamines, *anti*-acids, *anti*-hypertensives – prescribed by *anti*-doctors?) that interrupt chemical reactions causing distress. Toxic metals interfere far more. Our world is more toxic every year. Patients see "organ" doctors (for joints, heart, gut, skin) who ignore sneaky poisoning … so *your* health worsens by the day. Makes sense to treat the *cause* not just the *complaint*!

We'll let you in on some distressing secrets that your insurance company and your doctors have not heard. MRIs are rarely necessary for joint problems. Cortisone never helps joints heal. "Rooster-comb" injections gives brief comfort but rarely strength. "*Standing*" regular x-rays are essential to show sagging effects of gravity.

Rarely do neck or back problems require surgery – same for virtually *all* other joints. Knee "scope 'n' scrape" operations have been challenged as providing no better result than … *doing nothing*. (Except they get you closer to your next scope surgery and then the *next* one ... and then finally "joint replacement.")

Many of our patients have been (mistakenly!) told that their problem is so severe that it is "bone-on-bone" and they need "new plastic and new steel." (You don't get a joint *replacement* – you get instead a joint *substitute* made of plastic and steel.) Joyfully, they often improve dramatically with prolotherapy, natural injections that stimulate joints and support tissues to heal. (Dr. T has a bit of experience: he has treated all joints this way in many patients for 27 years.) Results in virtually any joint can be long-lasting and sometimes dramatic.

Regardless of which advanced technologies that we need to use to get the improvement you deserve, rest assured that Dr. T has long been recognized for producing results: comfort and capability in people who have suffered for years.

What are *you* waiting for? Didn't you hear that Simple Simon Says ... Take personal responsibility for your wellbeing:

Get out of your pain and get on with your life!^{SM}

Here's a **"stump the doctor"** question: In the *first* year of medical school, students learn how body processes *work*; in the *second* year, they learn how illnesses develop and how your body uses *inflammation* as the *very first step for healing* and repair ... So, **why** do they learn in the *third* year to prescribe **anti-**inflammatories that **block natural healing**? Those drugs just make problems feel a little less painful – but then your unrepaired joints can continue to hurt and limit your activities months (usually years) into your future. Does your doctor have a good explanation why anti-inflammatory medications (even aspirin) make any sense?

When life is your choice, failure is not an option.^{SM}

Find it *now* – Fix it *right!*

Ask Bobby

Bobby was just like so many local Texas heroes, a high school football player whose knee troubles began in 1960. Surgery in 1970 did more damage than help and he suffered constant pains since. Fluid swelling was drained several times over the years; a knee-wrap brace reduced his swelling and helped a bit with support. Walking, climbing stairs, standing for long periods – his life was looking more and more limited. Over 40 years of *un*successful treatments helped convince him to try our "stem cells" after hearing how this marvelous new treatment actually repairs injured tissues.

Guys are often worse than gals in complaining of pain with needles and Bobby lived up to the reputation. What surprised him, though, was how quickly he began to feel better. He almost boasts as his quality of life is improving: "I'm able to walk up a flight of stairs like a person should without having to pull myself up with my arms, one step at a time." Bobby is excited about the prospect of a pain-free life in his later years, something he had resigned himself to believing was never achievable.

Surgery is *never* your "last resort." If you need it, it's your *first* choice, get scheduled! If you don't need it, it's *not even on the list*. But … *what if* you were told you really need surgery by **someone who *does not know*** about the safe, effective, unique, and patented "stem cells" that we have come to rely on in our practice? Would you want to get "all the facts"? Don't you deserve to give your fully *informed* consent?

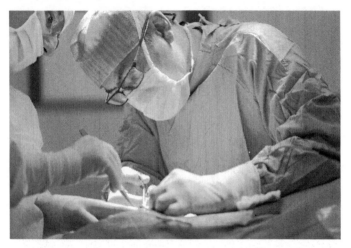

As we gain more experience with this patented, exceptionally powerful "stem cell" product, undoubtedly we will see where it can best be used – perhaps in place of surgery, perhaps to improve the results from surgery, perhaps to repair injuries to the point that they no longer need surgery that was earlier thought to be necessary.

Without a doubt, our special "stem cells" are producing results, reducing pains, improving sleep and exercise, and overall helping out patients to be more comfortable and more capable. *(Isn't that what it's all about?)*

When life is your choice, failure is not an option.℠

Find it *now* – Fix it *right!*

Choose Your *Health* Care
Like Your Life Depends On It

Too many times our choices regarding "getting better" are based on what pill or potion or operation that might *quickly* help you to "feel better."

Although we've had patients travel from all continents except Antarctica, the stories we hear sometimes are so sad:

"Couldn't you have an office in my part of Houston?" No.

"My local doctor says that he/she can do whatever you are doing." For which training programs has your doctor served as director and lead professor? What books has your doctor written? What lectures has your doctor given around the United States or overseas?

"I really don't want to drive that far or take that much time." Most everyone would be happy to drive to M.D. Anderson for cancer-care or to Texas Heart for specialized surgery … but often don't realize that enjoying daily comfort and capability as years go by can make a world of difference in life.

"My local doctor says his/her treatments work just as well as whatever you do." So please *help me to understand* … why are you *still* hurting, sick, and tired, and taking risky medications?

"I just don't want to have needles or take pills." Okay. How's *that* working for you?

"I'm waiting for insurance to pay for your services." Do you have a rocking chair and can you play checkers or BINGO, so you can pass the years?

"I really don't believe that your treatments could help me that much." Don't confuse you with the facts? The only one who still suffers is ... *you*.

"My husband/wife says that doctors like you just make phony claims and take everyone's money but you're not a 'real doctor.'" Come to our office, sit for a few minutes with our patients, hear their stories, decide for yourself.

"I don't want to spend that much – I have to keep my [rental houses][stock investments][CDs] [savings] for retirement." Are you aware that *nursing homes* charge about $4,000 or more each month – federal and state laws provide for them to lay claim to your assets until you have only a pittance left, apparently then you could qualify for Medicaid.

The *very worst* "excuse" that we hear is this: "I'm doing pretty well right now, I'll come see you when I need you." Nice thought. But *those* folks unexpectedly end up in the emergency room, which some have described as hopping on to the *medical* merry-go-round, with test after test and specialist after specialist. Expenses for drugs and surgery can mount up suddenly, insurance deductibles are enormous, continuing care devours your time and your money ... and then you don't have *any* funds or energy to seek effective *health* care *here*.

Just maybe ... taking time to learn how we might help you as much as we help most others

Find it *now* – Fix it *right!*

whom we accept for care makes sense. Comfort and capability allow you to experience a joyful life.

For details on Dr. T's professional background and expertise, check out his curriculum vitae at

www.healthCHOICESnow.com/CV   or scan ...

How did we choose the name for our website? To us, it's obvious: When you don't *know* that you *have* health choices *now*, then *you don't have any!* Our logo is an astronaut within a heart:

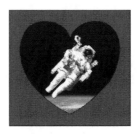

NASA pushes the limits of our understanding in all areas of science to design a spacesuit for survival in the hostile environment of outer space. We have never lost an astronaut on a spacewalk. Our body is the "suit" we depend on every minute of every day. At **Life Celebrating Health**, we push the limits of our understanding in all the biological sciences, nutrition, and pharmacology in order to help patients survive in the hostile environment of planet earth.

Because *health* is your greatest *wealth!*

Once again, honestly ask yourself these questions that are critical for your future:

When
does YOUR pain get in the way?

How long
have you suffered already?

How much longer
will you continue to suffer?

What do you fear
from more and more drugs?

What do you fear
from surgery ... *again?*

You want more than answers –
you want relief!

We're ready to help you *right now:*

DIAL 1-800-FIX-PAIN

When life is your choice, failure is not an option.℠

Find it *now* – Fix it *right!*

Ask Shirley

Years of low back discomfort have plagued Shirley off and on as an older adult. Even when not suffering with discomfort, she couldn't do much of anything without provoking an episode of extreme pain.

After seeing doctor after doctor and hearing experiences of friends, it's easy to become jaded and resigned that nothing is available to relieve deep and debilitating back pains. Despite her frustration, Shirley clung to the hope that maybe, just maybe, something could help.

We treated her low back with our special "stem cells." Within a week, Shirley was excited because her left leg and hip were no longer painful. She still notices some discomforts in her back but insists that she recovers quickly after rest with cold packs. After all these years of suffering, enjoying more comfortable days is a welcome relief.

For many people, there really are no words to describe the pain with which they live, day in and day out. Folks ask, "Hey, how are you today?" That's just a social greeting – because if you reply by describing your current pains, soon they show less and less interest. How can you blame them? They can't "fix" your problem and it seems to keep going on and on and on ... why don't you see a doctor and get it fixed?

After your storms of pain that feel like they will never end, God might offer you the reassurance He gave Noah: *"Whenever the rainbow appears in the clouds, I will see it and remember the everlasting covenant between God and all living creatures of every kind on the earth."* Genesis 9:16.

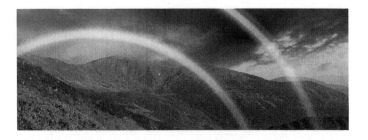

The National Institutes of Health are encouraged by the results of early investigations. Their research scientists conclude that stem cells might one day be used to repair damaged heart tissue, reducing the tragedy of cardiovascular disease, our #1 Killer. They caution that many more studies are needed to determine ways in which directing stem cells to develop might improve treatments for a wide range of diseases, such as macular degeneration vision loss, spinal cord injury, stroke, burns, diabetes, and others.

For now, we're thrilled with the results we have seen in our patients suffering with sports injuries and osteoarthritis (common wear-and-tear joint discomforts), among others.

When life is your choice, failure is not an option.℠

Poison Pills *Exposed!*

The risk of bleeding and death from **any** prescription *or even over-the-counter* anti-inflammatory pain and arthritis drug is well known, including "low-dose" aspirin, non-steroid "NSAIDS," and *all* cortisone-type medications. NSAIDs are the most widely used medications in the world, now listed as *Number 5* on the Top 10 Most Dangerous Drugs.

[In case you don't recognize the term NSAIDs: aspirin (*all* brands), ibuprofen (Advil, Motrin), naproxen (Naprosyn, Aleve), dozens of others: check with Dr. Google or your pharmacist. *Other* risks are related to acetaminophen – Tylenol.]

Medication-*caused* ulcers and other gut bleeding from NSAIDs kill many thousands of Americans yearly, a documented "side effect" in each drug brochure – not to mention their major risks for heart attacks and strokes, blood clots and pulmonary embolism, liver disease, kidney failure, and more. TV drug ads now race by like a blur, often ending with "and possibly even death." Many drugs nowadays carry similar warnings – but who expects to be the victim?

Known side effects – all potentially suffered by the *patient* not by the doctor.

Very early in my practice, I discovered *THE* answer: the phenomenal power of natural healing methods to reverse and even cure many problems that cripple us, steal our vitality, and even cause our death.

Filling your body with pills in the hope of feeling better? But you're not **made** of *medications*, you're made of your natural, living cells!

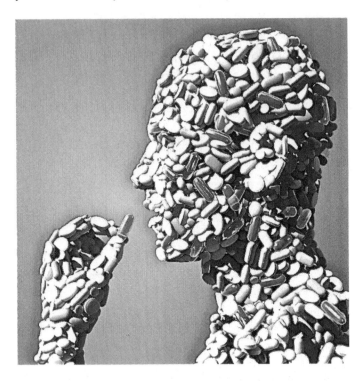

The FDA does insist that the ads rattle off a long, usually grim, list of potential side effects. But how could they do it without turning off "customers" (meaning: patients – *you!*)?

Well, a research study showed people commercials for two drugs that had similar side

Find it *now* – Fix it *right!*

effects and addressed the same health condition. One of the ads *rushed* through the risks, while the other didn't. People who watched the ad with the hurried narration had a much harder time remembering the drug's side effects.

Research has found that consumers absorb the most information when they can see people speaking rather than just hearing their voice. But sometimes all the positives are said by someone you can see and all the negative things and risks are said by an unseen off-camera voiceover. Did you ever wonder why *www.bad-drug.net* and 1-800-BAD-DRUG and *www.1800BadDrug.com* exist?

Joint "replacement" operations fare no better – remember, "new you" tissues (healing intended with our "stem cells") are *not* the result: instead, you get only a poor substitute, just "new plastic and new steel."

The chance of serious complications is about 1 in 50 in the first 30 days after operation. Studies show a markedly increased risk of death up to 3 months following joint replacement – many of these related to common heart/blood vessel diseases, lung diseases, even digestive disorders as well. Maybe dying doesn't concern you as much as the prospect of continuing ... *pain!*

Some follow-up reviews show 40% of patients are still suffering with persistent pain – often for *years*, even increasing as time goes by – *after* their successful knee "replacement." Their average pain rating is about "3 out of 10" but some suffer as high as "5" … which is about the same degree to which they were suffering *before* the operation.

Older patients are understandably at higher risk for surgery complications (or death) … but regardless of the hazards, pain can drive anyone to choose almost *anything*, hoping for relief. One often overlooked concern: younger, more active adults can face repeated operations, since 1 in 6 knee replacements will last only about 5 years, so "re-do" surgery is common. Those *later* operations involve greater risks of massive bleeding, longer anesthesia times, and infection, even failure.

Many people are hesitant to undergo operation – but their doctor insists that they have no other choice. What's sad is when such a trusted "professional opinion" is offered when the surgeon has little or even *no* knowledge of the remarkable results available with prolotherapy (natural injections into the joint support tissues, to turn on healing) or even beyond, with *our* "stem cell" product.

You might ask why specialist doctors don't actually know about these other treatments. The answers are simpler than you would expect:

first, the volume of information a doctor has to master is beyond imagination, so overlooking technologies not routinely in medical journals is easy;

second, when you already produce impressive results with "what you do," you have less incentive to look elsewhere for other alternatives; and

third, when the only tool you have is a hammer, all the problems you see look like nails – obviously all they need is to be pounded harder!

Find it *now* – Fix it *right!*

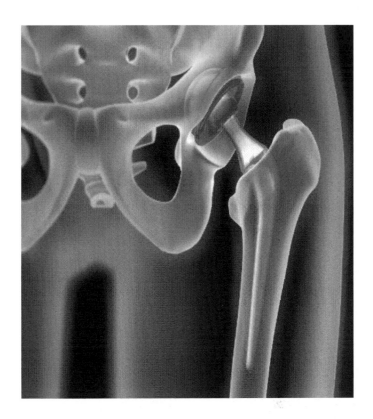

Choosing surgery to avoid those "poison pills"? One large study showed that half of "replacement" patients will begin taking a new pain drug during the first year after operation. Some 10% get new "nerve" drugs (side effects!); about 6% start new "narcotic" drugs (opiods – *addicting!*).

Younger operated patients – and any who have greater pain before surgery – often need more drugs. Alarmingly, about 1 in 6 knee "replacement" patients complain of "severe-extreme persistent pain" for years. Remember that the bones of your knee are amputated (cut off and discarded) in order to cement in your "new plastic and new steel" substitute. *What if … your earlier "knee pains" actually came from someplace else*, so that carving on your knee fails to resolve your discomfort?

While that idea might sound odd to you, think about this: ligament and tendon pain from strained/torn support tissues around or inside your knee. These soft-tissue problems can be easily misdiagnosed (missed!) by bone-and-joint doctors who operate on ... bones and joints. If your actual painful problem is *not* treated, you can continue to suffer for years. *"Close"* counts **only** in horseshoes, hand grenades, and shotguns.

Are you likely to get trapped into the addiction pattern of opioids (narcotic pain killers derived from opium poppies)? Over the past 2 dozen years, "legitimate" prescriptions have skyrocketed – not to mention "on the corner" purchases when long-lasting needs are desperate. This dramatic increase has one main explanation: our doctors are missing the reasons for our pains and, therefore, are failing to treat them successfully. ***Pain*** deserves *proper* treatment!

[In case you don't recognize the general term "opioids": fentanyl (Duragesic), hydrocodone (Vicodin), morphine (MScontin), oxycodone (Oxycontin), methadone, others.]

Long-term use (over 6 months) and higher doses can cause serious side effects. These include undesirable hormonal changes (especially in women),

Find it *now* – Fix it *right!*

weakening of your immune system (more risks for infections and cancers), worsening fatigue, brain fog, constipation, even the need for higher and higher dosages – *and addiction,* despite your best intentions. Misuse, overuse, and chemical dependency occur in about 1 patient in 4 "users" ... *you?*

Did your doctor warn you to be careful? Of course you are – but pain doesn't just **run** your life, eventually it **ruins** your life. Deaths from opioid overdose now *outnumber* those from car crashes and accidental or violent gun deaths combined. Other prescription and over-the-counter medications (as well as alcohol) can amplify the effects (and deadly risks) of opioids. News accounts often describe deaths where obviously the victim didn't expect *that* result from the drugs.

Is it finally the time to turn off your TV advertisements, avoid risky drugs, and look seriously at the benefits you might begin to enjoy with our safe, unique, and often very effective "stem cell" product?

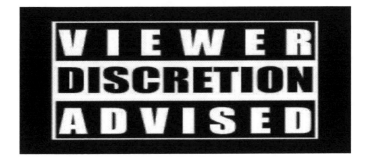

Facing the Facts About Pain

Pain is the most common reason for physician appointments in the United States.

Some 50 million Americans are suffering with pain.

About 1 out of 3 people are affected by pain.

About 140 million doctor office visits each year are for "pain management" or control – *not real relief!*

Pain can destroy your quality of life.

The Dalai Lama, revered head of Tibetan Buddhism, addresses the issue directly:

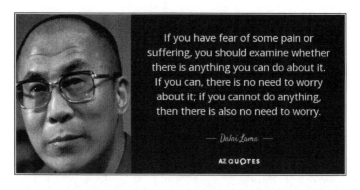

If you have fear of some pain or suffering, you should examine whether there is anything you can do about it. If you can, there is no need to worry about it; if you cannot do anything, then there is also no need to worry.

— Dalai Lama —

AZ QUOTES

So ... when you *can* do something about your pain, then there is no need to worry – *just do it!*

When life is your choice, failure is not an option.™

Ask Dan

Let's just say that Dan is "a big boy" –
actually he was a professional football player, except
for the injuries that kept him on the bench or off the
roster. The "spittin' image" of a "gentle giant," Big
Dan's picture would be right next to that definition in
the dictionary.

But Dan's life had become a bag full of
worries as adult-onset diabetes was rusting out the
blood vessels to his feet. Happily, toe amputations
had healed, because they often don't. But a
troublesome diabetic ulcer on the bottom of his right
foot simply would *not* heal. Blood sugar control:
great. Keeping weight off the foot: great. Visits to
the wound care center every 3 weeks for trimming
out the dead skin at the rim and deeper down: great –
but the wound stubbornly remained open despite the
best of medical care.

Ever hopeful for a solution, Dan found out
about a solution processed from the amniotic fluid
that surrounds and protects the growing baby in the
womb. His doctors said, "Sure, let's try it." The
surgery center manager said, "No way, not here."

Dan was able to get that healing solution
injected around the wound … and the sudden
improvement was startling. Within weeks, the
diabetic foot ulcer had healed – and Dan found a new
job, working with the amniotic fluid company,
sharing this exciting product with interested
physicians.

As happens with exceptional performers, Dan's successful reputation preceded him, and the company that developed the world's most unique "stem cells" recruited him to launch their patented product in late 2015. As a side benefit, those very cells have splendidly helped to restore the disintegrating support tissue and healing of new sole ulcers that resulted from walking across a hot driveway. What fool would walk across a hot driveway? One who *can't feel* the heat that is burning his skin. Diabetics suffer from decreased nerve sensations (neuropathy) and often fail to notice injuries happening.

Complicated illnesses often underlie what look like simple problems to the untrained eye. This simple fact is why a physician with specific expertise is essential for you to receive complete care, for your *whole* person.

Over time, non-healing ulcers and other **limb-** and **life-threatening** problems might need repeated special "stem cell" treatments along with personalized nutritional support, dietary changes, and other specialized programs. The goal is simple: create unexpected recovery by healing the support tissues and encouraging better circulation and nerve function, which means "life function"!

What do cells look like when they get "busy, busy, busy" repairing your tissues? Here's a microscopic picture, not easily obvious to "figure out" – but all *YOU* really care about are the results

Find it *now* – Fix it *right!*

you gain with less pain and more activity as your tissues are rebuilt!

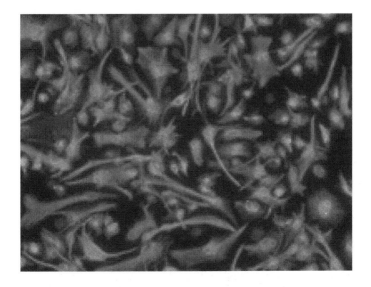

Looks like modern art you might even want to place on your wall. For now, let's "settle" for having these "busy-bodies" working enthusiastically inside, repairing your body injuries and restoring you to a life that is more comfortable and more capable.

Always remember that God put the healing instructions on the inside – all *I* have to do is find what is blocking you from getting better (remove it), find what you need but you're missing (provide it), find what switches need to be turned on (flip them on) – then step back and get out of the way! Our "stem cells" can help work that magic easily.

When life is your choice, failure is not an option.[SM]

Notes on Diabetic Foot Pain (Neuropathy)

Millions of people suffer with altered, uncomfortable, even painful sensations in their feet – or even loss of any feeling needed to have a warning sign. Diabetes isn't the only cause – blood vessel changes (peripheral arterial disease) can cause these nerve perception changes as well – and often both equally dangerous conditions occur together.

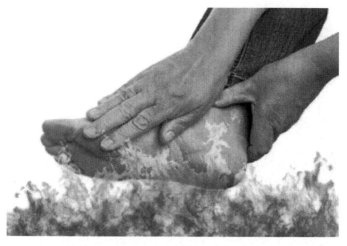

Our "stem cell" treatments might eventually show major improvements with neuropathy conditions. For the present, their most valuable effect is to allow and accelerate the repair of broken down, deteriorated, and often-infected structural tissues due to non-healing ulcers. Saving life and limb requires expertise far beyond just injecting cells.

Find it *now* – Fix it *right!*

Kick the Tail of the One-Trick Pony

Extreme changes in society, insurance programs, and medical practice itself have led not just to super-specialization but, sadly, to "clinics" that advertise and offer "quick results" for common problems. Single-focus quick weight loss and low-T (testosterone) clinics come to mind ... even others promoting stem cell treatments for whatever. Rather than helping find the solution *you need*, they assume that you need the solution *they have*. Whatever happened to doctoring the whole person? Not *there*.

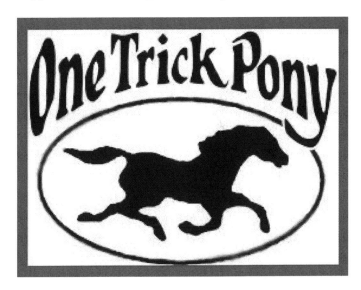

Other doctors are "like" Dr. T, they too have an M.D. (or D.O.) degree. Other offices are "like" ours, they too have assistants helping with treatments.

What sets us apart at **Life Celebrating Health** is our intense commitment to ... *your health*.

Here's a couple of outrageous examples to explain why our *comprehensive* approach can succeed when a narrow single-focus can fail. Do you know ... that a powerful antibiotic often prescribed for simple infections (where an older drug usually works just fine) can, literally, "melt" your joint support tissues, resulting in lingering pains and problems you never expected? Do you know ... that a medication commonly prescribed to lower cholesterol can cause muscle weakness and pains, even joint pains, problems that can remain years after you discontinue the drug?

Some folks would have you believe that your illnesses and your care are so simple that all you need to do is follow their program or get their injections. Others would have you believe that your illnesses and your care are so complicated that you "need" big words and fancy instruments and expensive pills or potions – none of which you are meant to understand. Dr. T insists on results and wants you to become an educated partner in your recovery, so that you can *continue* to feel better for years into *your* future.

Your job is to share your concerns and discomforts, **our** job is to figure out what is amiss and how to return you to a healthier, happier life. Some folks call us a "one-stop shop" for fixing most everything in your body. What surprises so many of our new patients is how quickly they can recover.

Dr. T is recognized as a world authority for his skill in diagnosing the root cause of problems

Find it *now* – Fix it *right!*

sometimes missed by major medical centers for years – then designing treatments that provide impressive improvements in just 3 months or so. That's why our simple slogan is … "Find it *now* – Fix it *right!*"

Our "stem cell" program is very helpful – but it is only *one* piece of the puzzle that you really need. You can't just "sign-up and pay," Dr. T has to review your condition and accept you into our care for whichever treatments will best help to solve your concerns.

Sadly, many people seek instant results (a "quick-fix") and they'll listen to almost anyone – trained physician or not – who crows a convincing promise. That's why internet ads for modern "snake-oil" miracles can make their promoters rich within weeks or months.

Many folks call our office, some shopping for particular treatments or bargain services. While they certainly have problems that need fixing, they impose their own ideas on what they need and what they are willing to "spend." There are clinics everywhere who will gladly cater to those people. Sadly, the "results" they provide might really "miss the mark." Manipulation of cells sucked out of your fat (belly or butt, even bone) by a clinic might interfere with their normal function in ways poorly understood. Some companies are marketing cells harvested overseas but relabeled as having been "sourced" here in America.

When there is no existing or effective treatment for a disease or condition, it is easy to understand why you might be blinded by hope and feel you have nothing to lose from trying something new, even if it isn't proven to the general medical community. Unfortunately, most of the unproven stem cell treatments for sale throughout the world carry very little promise of actual or lasting benefit and some can have very real risks.

A new phenomenon has appeared in 2016: advertisements promoting the use of stem cell "treatments" for a staggering number of diseases and injuries. A quick search of the internet brings up a long list of clinics offering what *appear* to be stem cell solutions for a wide variety of medical problems.

At **Life Celebrating Health**, we are very aware of how desperate you can be to find relief and feel better. That's why everyone who is accepted as a patient receives our intensely personal attention.

We definitely "do it different" from other offices. We have one question for you to answer: If doctors and patients keep repeating the same treatments that didn't work before, why should they expect different results with the next attempt? After all, how's *that* working for you?

Our testing and treatment approach is based on simple guidelines:

Safety – *first and always!*

Results – otherwise, why are we doing it?

And *then* …

Comfort

Convenience

Cost-consciousness.

Cost of care is *never* the major concern, since that would limit what might be the best approach or treatment to finally resolve your problems. We seek

Find it *now* – Fix it *right!*

to *safely produce results* for you the same way we would for our family: *that's* the **family standard of care**.

Correct diagnosis is critical; correct treatment is essential. Dr. T studies your history details, examines you (sometimes a patient is amazed that he actually lays hands on your body when other doctors didn't), and orders tests, all seeking to reveal the root causes of your problems.

Treating *where* your problems arise allows your body to do the natural healing that each and every one of us receives as a birthright from God. Sadly, many people unknowingly trade away this precious gift for a "bowl of porridge" that we now call drugs and surgery, and they often go through life miserable. [Remember that Esau sold his firstborn inheritance, his birthright, to younger brother Jacob for a bowl of lentil soup and bread, squandering his life and forever failing to appreciate his remarkable blessings from God. Genesis 25:29-34.]

Through extensive training and dozens of years helping patients heal, Dr. T has gained the skills to "juggle" the many (and often ignored, unseen, undiagnosed, untreated) factors that need his professional attention in order for your body to mend.

[Here's an exciting little secret: every year, Dr. T discovers newer "twists" to add to our already excellent programs. Even better: some of these discoveries consist of utterly novel approaches, never before introduced into practice. If you have a few hours, ask Dr. T to explain what startling information he has found out about yeast and fungus in the past 3 years.]

Back to juggling the many details that are essential for you to get results as expected – not just "stem cells" but much, much more involved with *whole* person (*wholistic*) medical and health care:

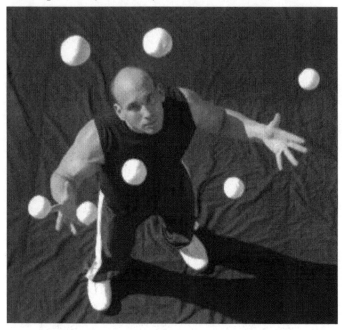

Remember that "close" counts only in horseshoes, hand grenades, and shotguns. Why trust your wellbeing to someone with less than world-class expertise?

We take our responsibilities seriously because pain doesn't just **run** your life, it **ruins** your life.

When life is your choice, failure is not an option.℠

Ask Joanna

Facing down her "golden years" at almost 65, Joanna agonized for many days each month with painful neck discomfort. Chiropractic adjustments gave relief for a few days at a time and prolotherapy injections (a natural solution to stimulate healing of strained, injured support bands) gave welcome comfort but never permanently.

Dr. T and the nurses spoke highly of the improvements they were seeing in patients with similar problems ... so maybe "stem cells" would be worth a try. Weighing the risks (hardly any) against the benefits (possibly a lot), the decision seemed obvious.

Joanna's treatment took just a few minutes. For two days, she was stiff and sore – and grumpy. To her surprise, the next day she realized that her headache was gone and her neck moved more freely and without much distress. As time went by, she felt more comfortable: sleeping was easier and more restful, activities were more enjoyable, her life had simply changed for the better.

Her husband observed that her eyes were no longer "tight" from the constant pain. Oddly, the "hump" at the base of her neck was softening, even disappearing. Some would think it's silly, but Joanna is thrilled that she can look up and turn her head enough to read signs.

After all these many years suffering with a painful neck, Joanna still has days where she is stiff and sore … but she notes these are further between and not excruciating like before. "Not being in constant pain has greatly improved EVERYTHING!"

Joanna's improvement shows something so valuable with stem cells: very few of our patients "need" more than *one* treatment. Could they *get* "more"? Sure – depending on how well your body heals, depending on other problems you have, even depending on your long term goals for comfortable activity.

After all, what price do people pay for comfort in their lives? ***Unless an effective treatment is found***, some folks turn to daily alcohol, others find that drugs and alcohol help blunt the pain, sadly a few choose addicting medications that change their lives in unspeakable ways. Everyone suffering with chronic or frequent daily pains experiences a change in personality: anger, fear, frustration, loss of patience, loss of enthusiasm, even loss of hope. Disrupting relationships and lives seems a terrible price to pay when relief might literally be within your reach.

In "the old days," we used to fear dying. Now, we fear getting sick. One major illness or injury – or lingering problems such as arthritis or other joint/muscle pains, that never go away – these can cripple your activities, paralyze your optimism, and literally steal your assets and bankrupt your family.

Injuries and aging changes can sneak up to the point where pain can steal any chance for restful

Find it *now* – Fix it ***right!***

sleep – and getting up from bed or out of a chair or out of your car can become a increasing challenge and a daily worry.

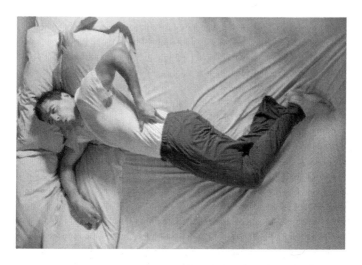

Inflammation chemistry is the powerful system used by your body to signal your stem cells to come clean up and repair the tissues. Inflammation is *painful!*, designed to force you to let the joints rest and recover. So … why haven't your own stem cells already gone to work to *solve* your problem?

So many people, as they get older, are suffering from "arthritis pains" in more than just one joint. Drugs can work everywhere – but their side effects can be worrisome, even deadly. Surgery, of course, can work on only one joint at a time. Our special, patented "stem cells" product can be easily injected to repair any inflamed joint.

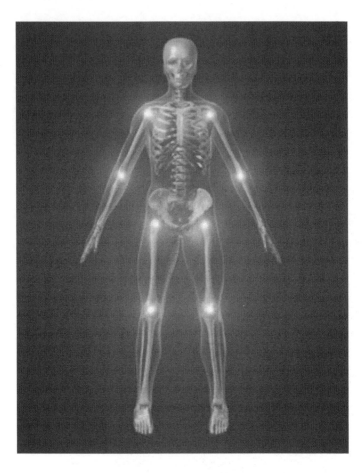

Take just a moment to consider the few dozen years of your life: growing up is fun and mostly has few problems; getting older is when we learn to ignore "stuff"'; as time goes by ... hasn't the time come to put out the painful flames in your body?

When life is your choice, failure is not an option.^{SM}

Find it *now* – Fix it *right!*

What Have We Learned Today?

✔ Injuries and illnesses cause inflammation.

✔ Inflammation is your body's signal, the first step required for healing: "Help, I have a problem and need repair over here."

✔ Inflammation can get "stuck" for a variety of reasons, then repair simply doesn't happen.

✔ Inflammation *hurts!*

✔ Pain limits your comfort and your capability.

✔ Drugs don't make healing happen.

✔ Drugs don't make pain go away.

✔ Operations don't make healing happen.

✔ Operations might make pain go away – *or not.*

✔ Pain that lasts for months or years – or even for the rest of your life – steals your happiness and wellbeing.

✔ Stem cells are born with you, hidden in your tissues, ready to respond to inflammation.

✔ Stem cells heal and repair injured tissues.

Because *health* is your greatest *wealth!*   49

✔ As you lead your life, your stem cells experience everything you do: stresses and toxic exposures, nutritional deficiencies, and so on.

✔ Adult stem cells, impaired by all the factors experienced by your other cells, become less and less able to perform needed repairs.

✔ When needed repairs remain undone, inflammation continues and even worsens, screaming for healing to happen.

✔ Our unique, patented "stem cell" preparation contains carefully selected and processed cells *and* needed cell growth factors and chemical support for maximum activity.

✔ When our "stem cell" product is injected into your inflamed tissues, they start working immediately to repair the problem.

✔ When your tissues are repaired, inflammation resolves because no signal is now needed to summon any help.

✔ When inflammation disappears, your pain becomes less and even goes away.

✔ When your pain goes away, you feel better and move more comfortably.

Find it *now* – Fix it *right!*

✔   When you move more easily, you have more capability to do what you want to do.

✔✔✔ *You win!*

You're hurting now and you haven't found anything that works like this, to make you more comfortable and more capable. You might be thinking to yourself, "I can't really believe that this could be true."

I know how you feel. I felt that way, too. And then I found out the facts about this *very* special "stem cell" preparation, way different than what I had read about with earlier products.

I found out quite by accident – just a chance conversation with a doctor friend who had just begun using these cells, which had finally become available only the month before.

And an accident was what drove me to try these "stem cells" for myself. I had ripped my knee apart in a (stupid!) fall 5 years earlier. Just minutes before our dinner conversation, I had reinjured my knee (white-lightning pain! *again!*) and I was limping badly.

After our discussion, of course I was more than mildly interested. But as my knee pains continued over the next few days, I became desperate and determined to try these "stem cells."

Going on faith, I ordered a vial and injected my knee. And my pain disappeared. Right then.

That day changed my life, forever and for the better. Now you know why I am so committed to helping my patients recover as well.

Our "stem cell" solution *deserves* the nickname of *"the package that performs!"*

When you were younger, recall that you could move comfortably and well. And you expected to do so for the rest of your life. Well, *today* is the *first* day of the rest of your life. Let's get crackin'!

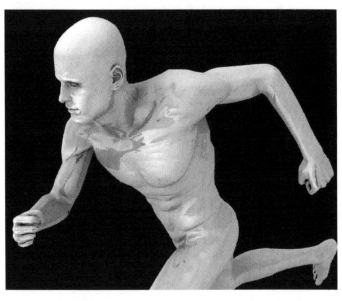

Aim for a purpose-driven life, one where you are empowered, passionate, enthusiastic, vibrant, vital, and robust. Choose to engage in meaningful and joyous relationships, fulfilling work, and cheerful play. ***Keep your eye on the prize!***

When life is your choice, failure is not an option.™

Find it *now* – Fix it *right!*

Safety First, Last, and *Always*

Hundreds of "clinics" have recently plunged headlong into the stem cell "business" across the country, despite serious reservations and little evidence for the safety and effectiveness of *their* procedures. Many of these "medical offices" are linked in large for-profit chains. These business models offer "doctors" the opportunity to join the franchise after attending a short seminar and purchasing expensive equipment for in-office harvesting (sucking your fat) and then manipulating your adult stem cells for reinjection into you.

The founder of Cell Surgical Network, plastic surgeon Mark Berman, has been quoted as saying "I don't even know what's in the soup [referring to the liposuction fat solution extracted from your belly or butt, maybe bone]," he candidly admits. "Most of the time, if stem cells are in the soup, then the patient's got a good chance of getting better."

If? *IF?!*

Sounds more like what the appliance salesman said when asked about a guarantee, *"You pays your money and you takes your chances."* We've heard charges as high as $25,000 for a single "treatment" (whatever "soup" that means) in a Beverly Hills clinic.

Now you understand why we deal in facts and an increasing body of clinical experience … ours.

Sufficiently convinced of their long-term safety for *me*, I can say without any reservation that I am thrilled to enjoy better comfort and capability, miracles for which I have long prayed as I have grown older. *Our* "stem cell" solution *deserves* the nickname of "*the package that performs!*"

This is "not your father's Oldsmobile," to borrow an advertising phrase boasting about all the engineering advances in their new model.

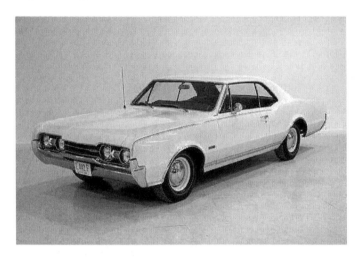

Remember that *ours* are "brand-new" cells, ready immediately to begin their healing work since your own cells have become lazy or inadequate. Studies have shown them to be safe and effective in repairing inflamed tissues, especially joints and other structures. When we talk about completely different, we want you to realize that *everything* is different due to their rigorous screening before collection, their processing at a regulated tissue bank: where and how they are obtained, how the specific active cells are separated out, how they are gently purified in order to retain vital life as well as the surface factors that help support and direct these cells to maximum performance when needed.

Everything is different? Think: *concept car!*

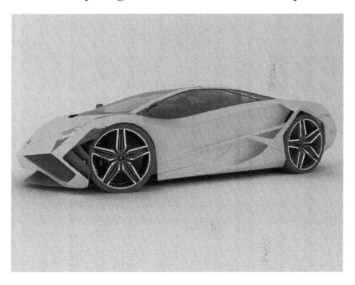

While it is unlikely that you'll ever be parking a futuristic Lamborghini in your garage, very likely you *will* be turning to this highly advanced, unique, patented and potent "stem cell" formula to help you become and remain more comfortable and capable as years go by. When you're suffering through your days and nights, sooner is always better than later.

Why not now?

When life is your choice, failure is not an option.℠

The miracle of healing and repair
proceeds with the innate intelligence
given to each of us by God as a
human birthright

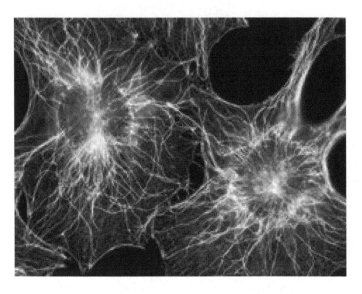

When I was training in surgery, the quiet
saying we learned early was this: If you ever want to
confirm that a surgeon believes in God, simply
observe him praying at a patient's bedside, over a
wound that will not heal.

As surgeons, we simply stitch together the
edges of an incision or wound ... but only God does
the healing. Thankfully He has given to us another
remarkable tool to promote and hasten our repair:
our unique "stem cells" that are fresh, young, and
ready to restore our wellbeing.

Find it *now* – Fix it *right!*

Who Wants To Live To Be 100?

Only folks who are *currently 99* and *feeling okay!*

We've seen some "advertising" for "stem cells" as an anti-aging or longevity or regeneration treatment. Honestly, that might be a major benefit, that topic certainly deserves further research.
While many claim they "want to live forever" – or maybe 100 or whatever ... what you really mean is that you want to live as long as you remain both ...

Comfortable
and
Capable.

For too many years, we've witnessed our seniors debilitated with aches and pains, where drugs provide little relief, longing for rest of any kind. Successful medical ***and*** health care, at the very least, keeps ***you*** living independently and free of misery or discomfort ... for a long time to come.

"The best doctor in the world is the veterinarian. He can't ask his patients what is the matter – he's got to just know." American actor, writer, and humorist "Will" Rogers might be onto something there ... but I haven't yet found a vet who will take care of *me!* So I have had to place my faith in ...

THE SECRET FORMULA:
2 C + 2 C = A+

Honestly, there are no secrets. Mastering success with your doctoring is quite simple when you take personal responsibility for your health care. *Your* responsibilities are summed up as " **2 C** ":

***C**urious* patient, ***C**ompliant* patient.

Plus the *doctors* you seek have obligations that also add up to " **2 C** ":

***C**ompetent* doctor, ***C**ommunicating* doctor.

The result is an **A+** in your life!

As a caring and curious physician, I was blessed that I "stumbled" early in my career to discover the immense power of natural healing. I have been driven to blaze a trail for patients *and* their doctors, leading to distant horizons of exceptional results with both *medical* **and** *health* care.

The secrets to "doctoring" are easy: study intently the emerging sciences, seek many details from your patients, ask probing questions and then listen intently, perform competent hands-on exams, and order and understand advanced tests that unlock the secret causes of inflammation, toxicities, deficiencies, and failing functions … so that they can finally be corrected rather than merely bandaged.

We specialize in pain *relief*
not pain *management*.

When life is your choice, failure is not an option.[SM]

Find it ***now*** – Fix it ***right!***

Just Waiting On *You*

We're standing by, ready and willing and able, whenever you choose to reach for a brighter, more rewarding future.

More than that, we see clearly that *our* job is "Just **Waiting On** You" – *we* know that *we're* here to **meet your needs**. Not to do tests or push pills or stick needles. Not to rush you in and out because dozens of others are piling into our lobby. Not to brush off your questions as we're leaving the room. Not to ignore your phone calls or faxes or emails when you really need answers.

YOU are here for results ... not for the experience. *We* are here to be **waiting on** you, just like the capable waiters that serve your every need and make your dining experience so enjoyable in the finest restaurants.

We were surprised to read this section, where **Dr. T dedicates this splendid booklet** to **us**, the ...

Awesome Staff of Life Celebrating Health

We're thrilled that he's the boss, developing incredibly successful diagnosis and treatment programs that we almost always see are helping our desperate and frustrated patients to get out of their pain and get on with their life ... *regardless* of the problems with which they have been suffering.

And like all great leaders, he absolutely relies on a well trained, enthusiastic, and reassuring staff to help meet the needs of those we serve.

Some folks are impressed with the "trappings" of impressive downtown buildings, high-rise elevators, expensive décor, fancy equipment, and the hushed formality of many medical offices.

What Dr. T values is … *us!* We show up each day bright-eyed and committed to make an amazing (occasionally unbelievable) difference, meeting the personal needs in *each* patient's life. Many of those who depend on us come from a long distance – and they cherish our single focus on meeting their needs. Our patients give meaning and purpose to our lives.

Our Senior Staff

| Cathy – 27 years | Rena – 27 years |
| Michelle – 13 years | Lucrecia – 6 years |

Our Rookies In the Dugout

Gabby – 2 years   Brooke – 2 years   Ebony – 1 year

So the only question for us to ask right now is …

"What may we do for *you* today?"

When life is your choice, failure is not an option.℠

Find it *now* – Fix it *right!*

We're ready to
make *your* life great again!

Dr. T – as he's been known since 1978 in our office – does "some" of the work … but we're thrilled to do all of the rest for you. Our staff of seven is lead by two of us who've been here 27 years each – our next junior assistant for almost 13 years. The others are "newbies," from 6 years on down. And we're all trained and excited and committed to helping him everyday: **"Find it *now* – Fix it *right!*"**

Send us your questions:
                    info@healthCHOICESnow.com
Fax us your questions: 281-540-4329
Call us with your questions: DIAL 1-800-FIX-PAIN

We work diligently to get you the right answers as soon as possible. *And* we invite you to come visit us face-to-face and talk with our patients too! We're easy to find: a 2-story red brick building right across the street from the Memorial Hermann Northeast Hospital in Humble, ½-mile south of Deerbrook Mall (FM 1960), just south of Tejas Toyota on the southbound feeder of US 59/I-69 in northeast Houston.
        You can count on our best efforts, always. We go home gratified each day that we had the joy, the honor, the privilege to help you ***get out of your pain and get on with your life.***^{SM}

Now for the good news: Dr. T researches and probes daily to introduce newer, outstanding treatments. We never have a dull moment, always learning and preparing to make all of *your* moments *better and better!*

But maybe *your* problems are *different …?*

Relax – most everyone is hesitant to get excited and hopeful when learning about a treatment they've never heard about the scientific facts before.

Yes, *we* know what conditions we help and about how much relief you can expect. We're one of the most qualified and respected offices in the country. We proudly share our experience with doctors around the country.

So … rather than let this incredible opportunity slip through your hands, just do this now: **call us** with your questions: DIAL 1-800-FIX-PAIN. **Send us** your x-ray or MRI or CT scan reports, write out just a brief note about what has been bothering you, how long you've been suffering, what you've tried but it failed to help. Dr. T will review your very real concerns and offer you genuine answers! (*No charge for this professional review and opinion!*)

Now is the time for you to pause – to close your eyes – to visualize how your life would look if you were to find healing with unexpectedly wonderful results. Could these "stem cells" actually provide such a result for you, too? With just a phone call, you could find out.

Find it *now* – Fix it *right!*

Full Disclosure: Dr. T is just a bit biased. You see, he has suffered with painful joints for almost 60 years and has had over 2,000 chiropractic treatments to keep him "almost" comfortable. He endured daily distress with a genetic condition rather like double-jointedness but more extreme, so he injured literally *every* part of his body, just usual living each day. Other treatments (prolotherapy to stimulate healing, which *we also do!*) certainly reduced his own discomforts over the past 27 years. Receiving our "stem cells" has been the miracle he long prayed for – and for which he is eternally grateful.

I praise You, for I am fearfully and wonderfully made. Psalms 139:14:

Hint: Gentle chiropractic – "low force, low velocity" – can help relieve neck or back discomforts far beyond what many people believe. So ... check it out!

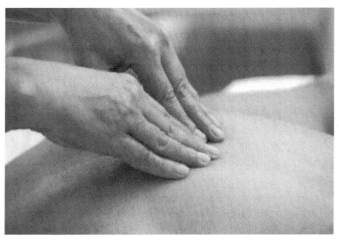

When life is your choice, failure is not an option.^{SM}

We have every reason to enjoy
when our patients find pain relief
from *our* commitment to
life ... celebrating health!

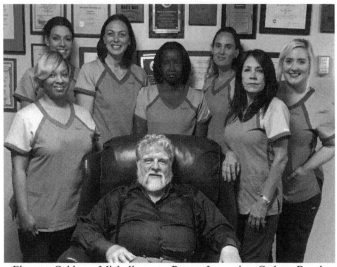

Ebony – Gabby – Michelle   Rena – Lucrecia – Cathy – Brooke

Dr. T

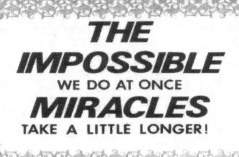

THE
IMPOSSIBLE
WE DO AT ONCE
MIRACLES
TAKE A LITTLE LONGER!

When life is your choice, failure is not an option.℠

Find it *now* – Fix it *right!*

Now Review the Impact of Pain in *YOUR* Life

You've taken the medications, you might have done physical therapy or even surgery. Maybe twice. But pains continue to steal your comfort and your capability – you are literally watching your life fade away while others go on.

Take a minute to **touch** the joint (or joints) that are causing daily or frequent discomfort. How long have you suffered? Do you remember the original injury? How did *that* feel back then? Did you have *any* idea that, years later, you could now be suffering pains that limit your life, your comfort, your capability?

Often we seem resigned to a false idea that aging is just "what happens." Aging is a *disease* that happens one day at a time. Our modern technologies can help restore your vitality, your enthusiasm, your activities in ways you might have long forgotten.

Take counsel in the science of the patented allograft ("stem cell") product we use, ethically obtained at scheduled C-section deliveries, strictly from the umbilical cord. Carefully separated from that "cord blood" are the active "mesenchymal" [multipotent connective tissue cells that can develop into the parts of multiple organs] stem cells, along with active cell factors. This science is *new* and is *now* available for you to enjoy the benefits.

People who know absolutely nothing about these latest advances are likely to be skeptical and discouraging to your interest in our "stem cells." The only answer is simple: get the facts, just the facts.

The warning in Proverbs 12:15 is so true at this important time in your life: The way of a fool is right in his own eyes, but a wise man listens to advice.

We make so many choices that we hope will bring us happiness. Sadly, "stuff" rarely meets our needs – but we're often willing to make those costly purchases. True joy is sleeping well, waking rested and happy, going through your days more comfortable and more capable. Science now offers you a precious choice: the patented, advanced "stem cells" product that we use … *the package that performs.*"

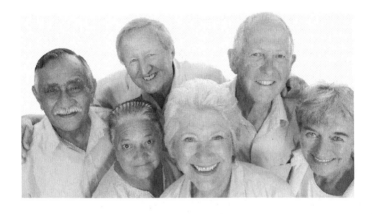

When life is your choice, failure is not an option.^{SM}

Headaches

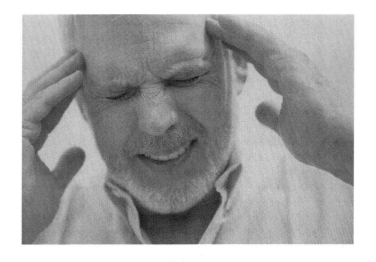

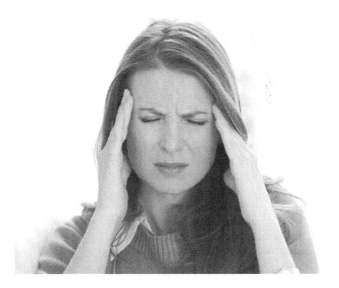

Neck Pains

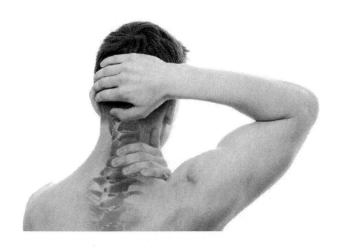

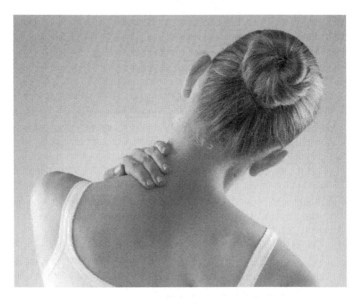

Find it *now* – Fix it *right!*

Mid-back Pains

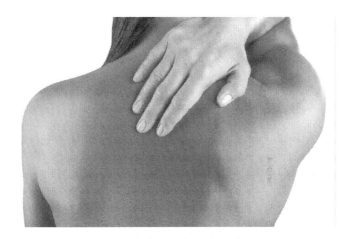

Low Back Pains

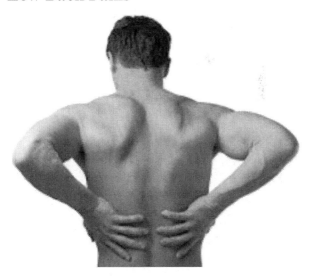

Because *health* is your greatest *wealth!*   69

Hip Pains

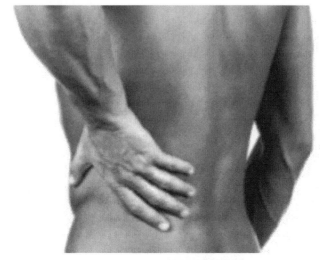

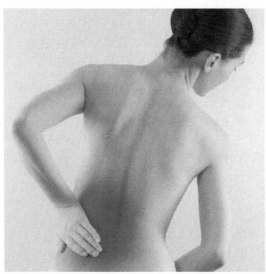

Find it *now* – Fix it *right!*

Knee Pains

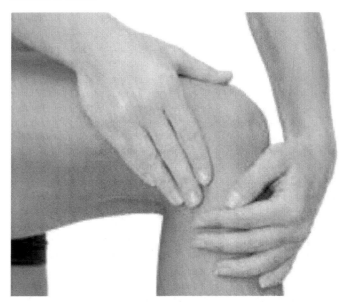

Ankle Pains

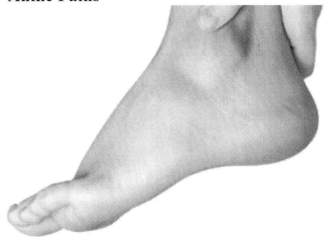

Because *health* is your greatest *wealth!*

Heel Pains

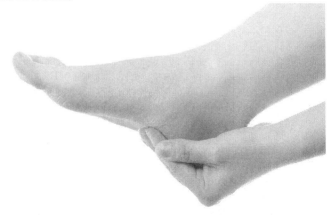

Foot Pains / Arch (Sole)

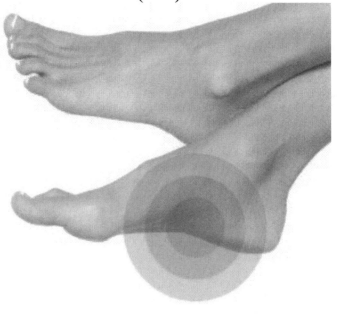

Find it *now* – Fix it *right!*

Foot Pains / Sole, Ball of Foot, Toe Pains

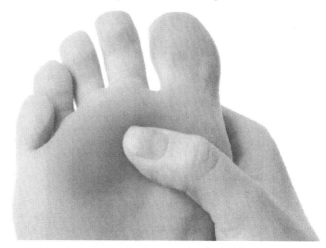

Especially Diabetic / Circulation Ulcers

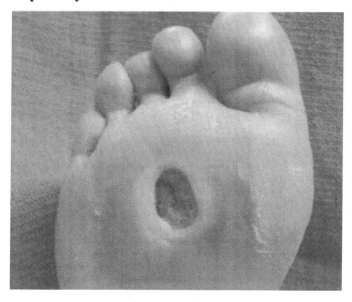

Because *health* is your greatest *wealth!*

Shoulder Pains

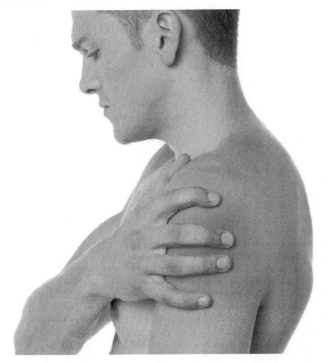

Elbow Pains

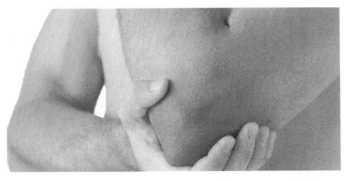

Find it *now* – Fix it *right!*

Wrist Pains

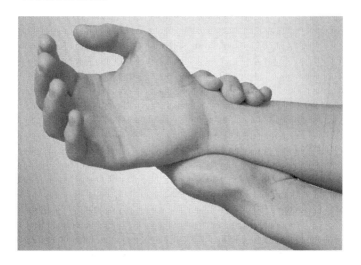

Hand Pains

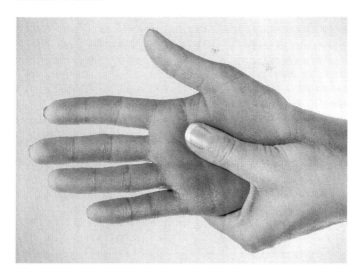

Because *health* is your greatest *wealth!*

Frustrating Pains with Jaw Joints (TMJ)

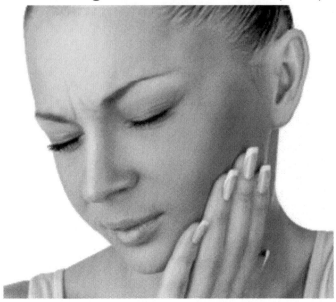

What About **YOUR** Joints?

These illustrations show you how many different ways that we suffer daily then through into later life. Sports injuries, accidents, car crashes, falls – the list is endless. Often we didn't go to the ER or even see a doctor "because it's not that bad." After a few days or weeks, you feel mostly "okay." But stretching or crunching support ligaments and tendons or even joint tissues themselves creates weakness that worsens over time. As we grow older, the "aches and pains" of ~~aging~~ *unrecalled injuries* grab hold and limit our comfort and our capability.

When life is your choice, failure is not an option.[SM]

Find it *now* – Fix it ***right!***

Are You Ready To Make the Call?

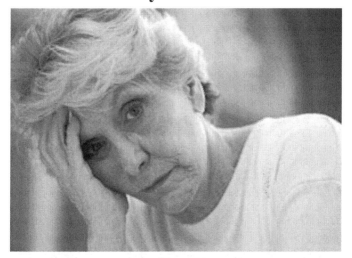

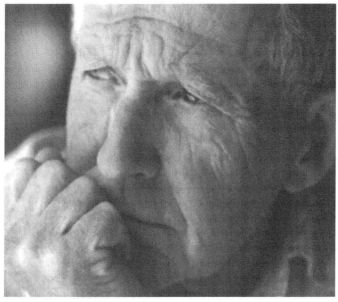

Because *health* is your greatest *wealth!*

DIAL 1-800-FIX-PAIN

Your only "cost" is just a few minutes ...

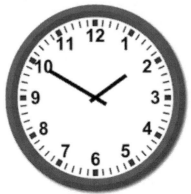

And what you gain could be *priceless!*

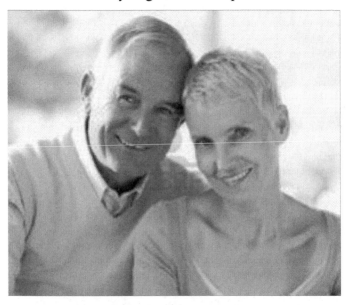

When life is your choice, failure is not an option.[SM]

Find it *now* – Fix it *right!*

Life Celebrating Health

9816 Memorial Blvd – Suite 205
Humble – Texas
DIAL 1-800-FIX-PAIN
www.healthCHOICESnow.com

What we do for you …

The easiest way to explain our services is simply that
we **"Find it *now* – Fix it *right!*"**

Correct diagnosis is critical – correct
treatment is essential! Dr. Trowbridge has trained for
45 years to look for and treat the cause of your
problems not just slap on another fancy Band-aid.
Sadly, many doctors don't have the time or perhaps
even the experience to recognize deeper reasons why
you are suffering … then to design safe, effective,
often natural solutions.

Respected for his incisive thought and broad
perspectives, Dr. T's accomplishments are
recognized in over 5 dozen volumes of ***Who's Who*** –
and by being named a Fellow of the American
College for Advancement in Medicine – and by
receiving the Distinguished Lifetime Achievement
Award from the International College of Integrative
Medicine.

Best-selling author of several books, Dr.
Trowbridge lectures across the country and around

the world. He has authored several invited articles on integrative treatments of cardiovascular disease for the *Townsend Letter* and on various topics for other journals and newsletters.

Dr. T has served as president, officer, or director of several professional associations, among these are the International College of Integrative Medicine, the International Academy of Biological Dentistry and Medicine, the American College for Advancement in Medicine, and the National Health Federation.

His devotion to patient education has resulted in several books, radio shows, CDs, and DVDs. Most notable is his million-copy best-selling Bantam Book **THE YEAST SYNDROME** – in some circles he's known at "The Yeast Doc." Soon to be published is **Mastering the Art of Success** with Jack Canfield of the Chicken Soup for the Soul series; Dr. T's chapter won the Editor's Choice Award. Another forthcoming book is ***Driven!*** with internationally acclaimed motivational speaker/author Brian Tracy.

Forthcoming in 2018 will be the flagship volume (on diagnosis and treatment of heart disease) in his new ***Doubt Your Doctor***™ book series, giving readers easy-to-understand guidelines by which to review whether their specialists are providing the care they really need. People have turned to Dr. Google in frustration; these books will help steer them in all the right directions.

Find it *now* – Fix it *right!*

Dr. T's present clinical research interests include exploring the best procedures for using our "stem cells" to help patients suffering with pain; diagnosis and development of treatment programs for unexpected/deep-seated fungal and parasite infections in a number of apparently unexplainable illnesses (cancer, leukemia, leukopenia [low blood counts], MS, sudden kidney failure, severe skin rashes/infections, and so on); improvement or control of atrial fibrillation rhythms by non-drug treatments; accelerated healing with natural prolotherapy (tissue growth stimulating) injections for patients with joint injuries, neck and back pains, and arthritis; and advanced treatment strategies to manage and prevent cardiovascular disease, especially congestive heart failure and recovery from heart attacks, strokes, peripheral arterial disease and gangrene, and diabetic ulcers and neuropathy.

We invite you to browse our website to learn more about the many treatment programs we offer to help you, your family, your friends:

www.healthCHOICESnow.com   or scan ...

Under construction/coming soon:
stem-cells-usa.com   or scan ...

Our new site will be a valuable resource for you
in coming months and years.

Here's our little secret: Right now, you can
download and print a *free* pdf copy of
Failure is not an Option from this webpage:

www.healthCHOICESnow.com/stem-cells   or scan

SPECIAL BONUS FOR OUR READERS:
Mention this booklet during your telephone
or in-person discussion with our
Treatment Consultants
to receive a certificate for a valuable benefit
to boost your recovery from pain.

When life is your choice, failure is not an option.℠

Failure is *not* an Option is published by
Appleday Press
P. O. Box 60899 – Houston - Texas
ISBN 978-0-9990112-0-1
ebook pdf download ISBN 978-0-9990112-1-8
Copyright at Common Law 2017 John Parks Trowbridge
First Printing May 2017 – Printed in the United States of America

This book is **not** medical advice but presents only general information. Nothing in this book should be understood to offer specific treatment for **any** individual. Presented herein are unbiased facts, solely the professional medical opinions of the author. All reasonable care has been taken by the author to provide these details accurately, and he does not accept any responsibility or liability for any reliance on the material presented. **Discuss any questions with your treating physician**. No commercial funding or sponsorship was sought or provided. The U.S. Food and Drug Administration (FDA) recognizes that the allograft cell product ("stem cells") used by Dr. Trowbridge are produced by a federally registered tissue bank that complies with HCT/P's and are regulated under the 1271 guidelines. Such products do not have a specific indication for use. They are intended for homologous (human) injection as determined by a skilled physician. Illustrations and photographs have been adapted from the public domain and are not known to be restricted from use in this publication.

Copies available:
DIAL 1-800-FIX-PAIN [349-7246]

Feel free to make copies to share with
your family, friends, coworkers, social club.
Commercial reproduction or distribution or use in any way
by any medical or health care provider or similar facility
is expressly prohibited without written authorization

We invite you to enjoy a book that has saved lives:
THE YEAST SYNDROME
Bantam Books Best-Seller 1986
All booksellers and e-book versions

Learn about other life-saving programs:
Life Celebrating Health
has over 50 CDs and DVDs
DIAL 1-800-FIX-PAIN
Because *health* is your greatest *wealth!*   83

Pages I want to share with friends:

_____

_____

_____

_____

_____

_____

_____

_____

_____

_____

_____

_____

_____

Proverbs 3:5-6: Trust in the LORD with all your heart, and do not lean on your own understanding. In all your ways acknowledge Him, and He will make straight your paths.

When life is your choice, failure is not an option.™

Find it *now* – Fix it *right!*

64319136R00048

Made in the USA
Lexington, KY
05 June 2017